VEGETABLES
PART-1
Nutritional and
Medicinal Value

Harshita Joshi

Table of Contents

Tables

Introduction

Consumption of vegetables in either cooked or boiled or raw form as a salad is a common routine in all the households. Most of the people consume vegetables in order to complete their balanced diet. Various types of vegetables are sold in the market to prepare a number of healthy and relishing dishes. It is also known to most of the people that these vegetables are very rich sources of nutrients especially vitamins, minerals and roughages. Some of the vegetables are very good sources of water too. We all know that these vegetables provide nutrition but it is rare to have thoughts about the amount of nutrition each vegetable is contributing to carry out the metabolic activities and regulatory mechanics of our body. Vegetables are considered as natural medicines that have healing properties and help in building up the immune system of the body. Very few people are discerning about the nutritive value of the vegetables they are consuming. It is also true that most of these common vegetables are easily grown by the home gardeners. The part one of the book details about the nutritive and medicinal value of all the common vegetables grown and consumed by a majority of the people. Some of these vegetables are highly valued as these are also used as cures against various irregularities of the body including heart disorders, diabetes, ulcers, asthma and rheumatism. One can easily lead a healthy and happy life with the addition of good amount of vegetables and fruits in their daily diet. In addition, most of the vegetables can be grown on the same piece of land as mixed crops. There is no need of special requirements while growing various vegetables in the home or kitchen garden. Expert health consultants also advise to consume about 400 gm of fruits and vegetables on a daily basis to prevent oneself from chronic diseases such as cancer and diabetes.

The annexure as the last section will give a clear idea of ideal amount of intake of vegetables on daily basis as well as amount of nutrients present in some of the common and easily grown vegetables.

Nutritional benefits of vegetables

A nutrient is a substance that is required by the body in any form to carry out its metabolic activities. These are proteins, vitamins, minerals, carbohydrates, fats and fibers. Vegetables are although low in fats and carbohydrates but very rich sources of vitamins, minerals, fibers and play effective roles in the regular functioning of the body. Vegetables are generally consumed as an additional dish along with staple diet either in cooked or raw forms but in some areas of the world, tuber vegetables are also consumed as a staple food. These are generally richer and inexpensive sources of nutrients. The medicinal properties of the vegetables have been known since ancient times and various ancient literatures also mention about the use of vegetables to cure lethal diseases.

Vitamins and Minerals

Vitamins

Vitamins are compounds used to maintain and regulate the body mechanism even if consumed in small amounts; however the requirement increases with increase in age. The main functions of vitamins are regulation of body processes, tissue building and body metabolism. These are categorized into water soluble and fat soluble vitamins. Water soluble vitamins comprise of Vitamin B complex and Vitamin C whereas fat soluble vitamins are Vitamin A, D, E and K.

Vegetables rich in vitamins

Almost 95% of the vegetables are rich sources of both fat and water soluble vitamins. Most of the vegetables contain appreciable amounts of Vitamin A, Vitamin E, Vitamin K, Vitamin B-complex and Vitamin C.

Vitamin A

Vitamin A is also known as Retinol and as the name indicates, it is required by the body mainly for healthy eyes and vision. The nutrient also strengthens the immune system of the body, keeps teeth, tissues and skin healthier. It is generally present in animal products however many vegetables also contain appreciable amounts of Vitamin A. All leafy vegetables, cabbage, carrot, lettuce and sweet potato are considered as richer sources of Vitamin A. Carotenoids are another form of Vitamin A that is mostly present in fruits and vegetables. The table details the vegetables that are rich sources of Vitamin A and can be grown easily and at any place in the kitchen garden. In order to save the space, roots crops are generally advised to plant on the ridges.

Table 1: Vegetables rich in Vitamin A

S.N.	Type of crop	Vegetables
1	Root crops	Carrot, radish, yams
2	Tuber crops	Sweet potato and potato,
3	Cole crops	Cabbage, kale, cauliflower, Brussels sprouts, broccoli and knolkhol
4	Bulb crops	Leek and small amounts in onion
5	Cucurbits	Musk melon, pumpkin, bitter gourd, ridge gourd, all squashes, cucumber, snake gourd, round gourd and pointed gourd
6	Leafy vegetables and salad crops	Lettuce, celery, beet leaf, spinach, fenugreek, amaranth
7	Legumes	Peas and French beans
8	Fruit vegetables	Chilies, capsicum, brinjal, tomato
9	Other vegetables	Okra, asparagus,

It is advised by all the health practitioners to have ample quantity of vegetables containing Vitamin A to overcome skin related irregularities, weak immune system and night blindness.

Vitamin E

The main function of Vitamin E is to strengthen the immune system and cardiovascular system of the body. It also has strong

4

antioxidant properties and effectively protect against heart diseases and cancer. Vitamin E is mostly present in vegetable oils, nuts and whole grain products and less in vegetables like green leaves. Other sources of Vitamin E in vegetables are broccoli, taro, pumpkin and asparagus.

Vitamin K

Vitamin K is also a fat soluble vitamin the major role of which lies in blood clotting. In addition, the vitamin also helps in protecting against heart diseases and cancer. The nutrient also assists in the formation of proteins for kidneys, blood and bones and is also protective against osteoporosis as well as external wounds.

Table 2: Vegetables rich in Vitamin K

S.N.	Type of crops	Vegetables
1	Cole crops	Kale, collards, broccoli, cabbage, cauliflowers and Brussels sprouts
2	Leafy vegetables	Spinach, mustard, parsley, lettuce
3	Other vegetables	Okra, leek, peas, asparagus and artichoke

Vitamin C

Vitamin C or ascorbic acid functions as an outstanding source of antioxidant. It is a water soluble vitamin that keeps the bones, teeth, gums, hormones, collagen and blood vessels healthy and also helps in absorption of iron and calcium. It also helps in strengthening of the immune system of the body.

Table 3: Vegetables rich in Vitamin C

S.N.	Type of crops	Vegetables
1	Solanaceous crops	Tomato, chili, capsicum, brinjal and potato
2	Cole crops	Cauliflower, cabbage, knoll khol, sprouting broccoli and Brussels sprouts
3	Root crops	Beet, turnip, radish, a small amount in

		carrots
4	Bulb crops	Onion, garlic and leek
5	Legume crops	French bean, cowpea and hyacinth bean
6	Cucurbits	Bitter gourd, musk melon, round gourd, pointed gourd, and small amounts in cucumber, pumpkin, bottle gourd and ridge gourd
7	Green leafy vegetables	Salad crops such as lettuce, parsley, spinach, beet leaf, fenugreek, amaranth, rhubarb and mustard
8	Other vegetables	Peas, lady's finger, sweet potato, tapioca

Vitamin B-complex

Vitamin B complex contains B1, B2, B3, B5, B6 and B9. The functions of all the vitamins are more or less similar with some peculiar differences that are detailed below-

Vitamin B1

Vitamin B1 or Thiamine is required by the body for production of energy along with carrying enzymatic reactions. The vitamin also helps in proper functioning of muscles and nerves. In addition it also facilitates production of fatty acids in the body.

Vitamin B2

Vitamin B2 is an important nutrient that is required for carrying enzymatic reactions, healthy vision, and better health of skin and hair, and energy metabolism. Additionally, the vitamin also reduces headache and migraine. Sometimes it also functions as an antioxidant and activation of Vitamin B6 and Vitamin B4.

Vitamin B3

Vitamin B3 is also required for facilitating enzyme reactions, better health of skin and nerves, and digestion. The vitamin also helps in lowering down the cholesterol level in the blood and subsequently reduces the risk of heart attack.

Vitamin B5

Pantothenic acid or Vitamin B5 is essential for proper functioning of adrenal gland, and metabolism of carbohydrates. It also helps in the production of bile acids, red blood cells, cholesterol, fat and hormones.

Vitamin B6

Also known as Pyridoxine, the vitamin is essential for metabolism of fats and proteins and production of red blood cells and neurotransmitters. Additionally the vitamin is also required for proper functioning of estrogen and testosterone hormone in the body.

Vitamin B12

Cobalamin or Vitamin B12 is important for the synthesis of nucleic acid (DNA and RNA), production of red blood cells and carrying enzymatic reactions in the body. As a medicinal compound, it is used against asthma, male infertility, heart disorders and cancer. It also functions in energy metabolism.

Biotin

Biotin is also required by the body for the synthesis of amino acids, glycogen as well as fat fibers. One of the important components of Vitamin B family, biotin is important for replication of DNA and maintaining better health of nails and hair.

Table 4: Vegetables rich in Vitamin B complex

S.N	Vitamin B	Vegetables
1	Vitamin B1	Peas, asparagus, okra, beans, celery
2	Vitamin B2	Winter squash, sweet potato, peas, broccoli, Brussels sprouts, asparagus and amaranth
3	Vitamin B3	Okra, artichoke, French beans, peas, squashes, pumpkin, sweet potatoes
4	Vitamin B5	Lima bean, pumpkin, okra, squashes, French beans, Brussels sprouts
5	Vitamin B6	Spinach, capsicum, turnip, squash,

		garlic, mustard leaves, tomatoes, beans,
6	Vitamin B12	Spinach, potato, asparagus, broccoli, legumes
7	Biotin	Soybeans

Folic Acid

Folic acid is another name for Vitamin B9. Like other vitamins Folic acid also helps in converting food to energy. It is present in wide sources of vegetables and sometimes also functions as a supplement if added to other compounds. The vitamin plays an important role in synthesis of nucleic acids and proper functioning of mental and emotional health of the body. With Vitamin B 12, folate helps in making red blood cells and proper functioning of iron, as well as controlling metabolism of amino acids. A recommended quantity of folic acid on daily basis helps in slowing down the progression of hearing with increase in age. It is must for pregnant women to consume vegetables rich in folic acid in order to prevent birth related defects in their children. Other important functions of folic acid are protection from cancer, heart diseases, depression and degeneration of body due to increase in age, memory loss and osteoporosis.

The major sources of folic acid are cereals, vegetables and fruits. Vegetables are one of the richest sources of folic acid. All dark green leafy vegetables, spinach, turnip, mustard, beet, cole crops, and legumes are very rich sources of folic acid.

Table 5: Vegetables containing Folate

S.N.	Type of vegetable	Vegetables
1	Green leafy vegetables	Beet, spinach, mustard, turnip greens and lettuce
2	Legumes	Kidney beans, lima beans, soybeans, peas and cowpea
3	Cole crops	Brussels sprouts and broccoli,

| 4 | Root vegetables | Carrot and turnip |
| 5 | Other vegetables | Asparagus and tomatoes |

Deficiency of nutrients

A healthy body requires adequate amount if nutrients for proper functioning of all the organs and for that it is important to consume recommended amount of food on daily basis. While lack of any of the nutrients imbalances the functioning severe deficiency of any of the nutrients is fatal. A deficiency in a body is defined as the lack of any of the essential nutrients leading to malfunctioning and malformation of organs and ultimately affects the growth and development of the body. Hence balanced consumption of all these essential nutrients is required for maintaining a healthy body.

Deficiencies caused by the essential nutrients resent in vegetables

Vitamin A

The deficiency of Vitamin A is very common in developing countries where the diet lacking sources of Vitamin A causes night blindness, drying of skin and eyes. The growth also retards due to the deficiency of this vitamin.

Vitamin D

The diet insufficient in Vitamin D causes rickets or weakening of bones in children and osteomalacia or softening of bones in adults. The deficiency also results in osteoporosis in adults. Other imbalances that occur due to the deficiency of Vitamin D are decaying of tooth and weakening of muscles.

Vitamin E

The deficiency of Vitamin E in the body results in unhealthy retina of the eye, weakening of muscles and sensory nerves. In addition other symptoms of the deficiency include in lack of coordination and balance.

Vitamin K
Vitamin K is essential for blood clotting hence the deficiency results in easy bleeding of gums and nose. It also results in blood while urinating or heavy menstruation and ultimately high loss of blood.

Vitamin C
The deficiency of Vitamin C causes scurvy where the symptoms include bleeding of gums, pains in joint, swelling, loss of hair and tooth.

Vitamin B
The deficiency of Vitamin B1 causes beriberi, where the major symptoms include improper functioning of muscular, nervous, cardiovascular and gastrointestinal system.

A diet inadequate in Vitamin B2 causes swelling and redness of mouth, lips, tongue and skin. In addition it also decreases the count of red blood cells in the body.

The deficiency of Vitamin B3 or Niacin causes Pellagra. The major symptoms of the deficiency are identified by rashes on the skin, dementia and diarrhea. The more severe case of the deficiency leads to death.

The deficiency of Vitamin B5 is only identified on the basis of symptoms of malnutrition. In most of the cases, the symptoms of this vitamin include fatigue, headache and feel of burnings in hands and feet.

The common deficiency symptoms of Vitamin B6 are depression, improper functioning of immune system and sores in mouth however in most of the cases the deficiency is not identified.

Common deficiency disorders due to lack of Vitamin B12 in the dies are loss of appetite, anemia, constipation, and depression.

A diet lacking Biotin mostly produces symptoms such as red rashes on eyes; mouth, etc., improper immune system, depression and laziness.

Folic acid or folate deficiency shows symptoms like diarrhea, improper immune system functioning, weakness, fatigue and headaches.

Minerals

Minerals are the compounds present in body cells. Minerals are required by humans as well as plants to regulate the fluid of the body, help in building tissues of the body and growth and development. Plants are considered as one of the important sources of minerals as these are also absorbed by the plant itself to carry out its metabolism in addition to growth and development. Some of the minerals also help in absorbing other nutrients required by the body. Calcium, Iron, Zinc, Iodine, Copper, Fluoride, Phosphorus and Manganese are some of the main minerals vital to both growth and functioning of the body although required in trace amount in combination with other compounds.

Calcium

The mineral plays a very important role in maintenance of bones and teeth and their development as well. Blood clotting, nerve impulse and muscle contraction, protection of bones from thinning are some of the other major functions of Calcium however excess of this mineral is also not suggested.

Table 6: Vegetables rich in Calcium

S.N.	Type of vegetable	Vegetables
1	Cole crops	Kale, broccoli, cauliflower and cabbage
2	Green leafy vegetables	Mustard, spinach, amaranth,
3	Bulb crops	Garlic, onion and leek
4	Legumes	Peas and all beans
5	Root crops	Carrot, turnip, radish and beet
6	Other crops	Okra, tomatoes, colocasia, tapioca, yams, artichoke, and potato

Phosphorus

Phosphorus is an essential component of bones, teeth, ATPs as it also plays an important role in the formation of high energy compounds and various nucleic acids. As the mineral is also required by the plants in higher amounts for their growth and development, almost all the vegetables are very rich sources of this essential mineral.

Iron

The mineral is essential to transfer oxygen between the tissues. In trace quantity, it is required for many proteins and enzymes especially hemoglobin and myoglobin proteins that carry oxygen in the blood. The red color of blood is only due to presence of iron in it. Iron is also required for synthesis, packaging and uptake of neurotransmitters[1] and later their degradation into iron containing proteins. The deficiency of iron leads to anemia while excesses results in haemochromatosis[2].

Dark green vegetables such as beet leaf, spinach, mustard leaves and fenugreek are very rich sources of Iron. In addition, beans such as cowpea, hyacinth beans and French beans are also considered s appreciable sources of iron. A good amount of iron is also found in peas, salad vegetables, cucurbits and sweet potatoes. Solanaceous crops, cole crop, root crops artichoke and rhubarb also contain iron in trace amounts.

Copper

Copper helps in absorbing iron from the gastrointestinal tract and the formation of red blood cells along with iron. It also functions as an antioxidant. Like iron, copper is also an important component of enzymes. The mineral is also necessary for the formation and growth of bones however it is required by the body in trace amounts and the excesses lead in negative liver functions.

---

[1] The chemicals that allows that act as messengers to communicate and also connect the brain with the body
[2] An inherited disorder in the body resulting in absorption of too much iron in the body

13

Solanaceous vegetables like brinjals and tomatoes, carrots, beans, peas and green leafy vegetables are sources of copper.

Manganese

Manganese is actively involved in the formation of amino acids and enzyme activation. The mineral is an important component in the formation of bones and functioning of muscles and nervous system of the body. It is also one of the essential parts of enzymes involved in the formation of urea and breakdown of carbohydrates and cholesterol. Although manganese is also required in trace amounts and deficiency is also not visible but like other minerals, it is also vital in carrying out the regular activities of the body.

Some of the richest sources of manganese are spinach, mustard, garlic, soybean, French beans, brinjal and squash.

Zinc and Iodine

Zinc is an essential mineral required by many enzymes of our body to carry out their functions properly. It strengthens the immune system, tissue and wound repair and also helps in clotting of blood. The mineral is also required for synthesis and digestion of proteins, regulation of sugar levels in our blood as well as cholesterol. Iodine on the other hand is essential for the synthesis of thyroid hormone and protects against goiter. Sometimes, the mineral also acts as an anti-oxidant.

Green peas, spinach, asparagus and beans are good sources of zinc while sea vegetables contain appreciable amounts of iodine. Mostly the deficiency of iodine is overcome by the addition of iodized salt in the daily diet.

Other than these essential minerals, vegetables also contain minerals like sodium, chlorine, potassium, sulfur and magnesium that directly or indirectly help in carrying on the regular functions of the human body.

Deficiency of minerals

Like plants, humans also require essential minerals to carry out various processes in the body and lack of any of the minerals produces the deficiency symptoms that on later stages, if not cured timely becomes fatal for the health. The deficiency symptoms of minerals shown by humans are not so prominent and easily identified as compared to plant however a better understanding of the common symptoms gives effective results for curing the disorders. This section gives a glimpse of some of the easily identifiable symptoms that are produced by the body due to deficiency of any of the minerals.

Calcium is an essential component for the formation and maintenance of bones and teeth and the deficiency of this mineral is identified by weakening of bones, rickets in children, tooth decay and pains in legs and back of the body.

Poor appetite, weakness, osteoporosis, kidney stones, depression and anxiety, and high blood pressure are some of the commonly identified symptoms of deficiency of magnesium in the body. Similar deficiency symptoms are shown if the body is deficient in phosphorous. Other symptoms also include anemic appearances, weaknesses in muscles, poor immune symptoms etc.

Iron, copper, manganese, zinc and iodine are trace elements and are required by the body in very small amounts however the deficiency of any of these mineral leads to attack of various disorders.

The deficiency of iron is more common in women and vegetarian and the common symptoms produced by the body due to its deficiency are anemic appearances, headache, increase in heart rate and breathing, poor immune system, yellowing of the body and severe headaches.

The deficiency of copper in human body results in decrease in count of white blood cells, improper skin pigmentation and growth impairment in children.

Zinc deficiency is common in malnourished children and women and the symptoms include diarrhea, loss of appetite, rashes on skin, weakness in sensing, night blindness, weak immune system etc. The deficiency of iodine in the body reduces production of thyroid hormone resulting in goiter. Other symptoms of the deficiency include fatigue, reduced growth and increase in weight.

Other important components

Fibers

Dietary fibers are present in almost all of the vegetable and fruit crops which help in protecting the body in several ways some of which include constipation, diabetes, health, weight, and heart diseases. Unlike animals, human body does not contain enzymes that can digest fibers or roughages however these are important for a healthy body in terms of helping in digestion and maintaining the weight. Vegetables contain both soluble and insoluble types of fibers. A soluble fiber is dissolvable in water and helps in lowering the cholesterol level as well as glucose level in the blood. On the other hand, insoluble fibers are not dissolved in water but helps in movement of waste material through the digestive system and help in relieving from constipation.

The major sources of soluble fibers are vegetables such as beans, peas and carrots and vegetables that contain the good amount of insoluble dietary fibers are cauliflowers, potatoes and green beans.

Antioxidants

Free radicals in the body are produced when the body undergoes digestion, exposure to smoke or radiations. These free radicals damage cells and also disrupt the body and cause cancer and heart diseases. Antioxidants protect the body from free radicals. All the vegetables that contain Vitamin A, Vitamin E, Vitamin C, and Beta Carotene have antioxidants.

Table 7: Some vegetables having anti-oxidant properties

Sources	Examples of some Vegetables
Vitamin A	Carrot, spinach, Brussels sprouts, squash, broccolis, tomatoes and sweet potatoes
Vitamin E	Salad vegetables and vegetable oils
Vitamin C	Potatoes, broccolis, tomatoes

Water

Water helps in performing various vital functions in the body. The major function of the compound is to distribute nutrients to the body cells. Later is also helps in movement of body wastes after digestion of body in the form of faeces and urine in other words, functions as a medium to carry out metabolic reactions in the body. With the removal of wastes all the toxins that are harmful for the body get removed. Other vital functions of water include regulation of body temperature by facilitating release of extra heat from the body, and also work as a lubricant around the joints. Because of these essential roles in the body, it is advised to drink a recommended amount of 3-4 liters of water on daily basis, the irregularity of which will cause serious disorders.

Water is also a medium for growth of the vegetables that performs similar functions as in humans. Hence all vegetables contains water however on an average the highest amount of water is present in cucurbits. Therefore it is always recommended to eat watermelons and cucumbers to cool the body during scorch summers. The table in the end details the percentage of water present in each vegetable.

17

Medicinal benefits of vegetables

The practice of curing diseases using natural sources is very old which is well described in various ancient literatures. Vegetables are considered as one of the best sources to prevent one from many types of illnesses ranging from small allergies to deadly cancer. Regular intake of vegetables at recommended amounts will help in leading a healthy life. The chapter here details about vegetables, the regular consumption of which will help in staying away from wide ranges of diseases. All types of vegetables help in protecting the human body either directly or indirectly by fighting with disease causing pathogens[3]. It is already discussed earlier that these vegetables are very rich sources of nutrients especially vitamins and minerals that help in keeping a regular check on the metabolic processes[4] of the body. Even in rural areas that are yet to be accessed to nearby medical institutions, use traditional methods to cure diseases.

Important vegetables and their role in curing the diseases

Solanaceous vegetables

Brinjal, tomato, chilies, capsicum and potatoes are the important vegetable fruits of the Solanaceae family. Each of the fruit vegetable plays an important role in providing essential minerals and vitamins to the body that later helps in preventing various ailments.

---

[3] An agent that causes disease
[4] The catabolic (break down) and anabolic (synthesis) processes in the body

Potatoes

Potatoes are good sources of energy; also contain Vitamin A, Vitamin C, potassium, iron, magnesium and sulfur in appreciable amount. Other important minerals present in the tuber are iron, sodium, calcium and chlorine. The good amount of potassium helps in maintaining the blood pressure to the normal. It also possesses anti-cancerous properties. Another important role of potatoes is curing various disorders of the stomach such as hyperacidity and gastritis. The tuber is a good source to cure skin rashes and also as a bandage against burns.

Egg plant or Brinjal

It is a myth to consider brinjal as a poor nutritive vegetable now. Brinjal is a very important vegetable that helps in controlling the diabetes, protection to the brain and heart, assisting in digestion, and weight loss and stomach problems like flatulence. This vegetable fruit has anti- bacterial properties and also contains a good amount of potassium, phosphorus and Vitamin A. Brinjal also acts as a cure for hypertension, cancer and rise in cholesterol level in the human body.

Tomatoes

Tomato is the most important fruit vegetable of all the other Solanaceous crops. It is the most common fruit vegetables and an important ingredient in all the recipes. Tomatoes are excellent anti-oxidants; contain higher amounts of vitamins and minerals. The fruit contains lycopene that is an anti-oxidant and anti-cancer agent which also gives the red color to it. This agent helps in regulating blood circulation, strengthening immune system, preventing cancer and other tumors as well as exercise induced asthma. The other medicinal properties of tomatoes also include cure against rheumatism, remedy for uric acid and aiding in proper functioning of liver.

Peppers

The presence of alkaloid compound capsaicin makes chilies an important Solanaceous fruit vegetable that help in fighting against carcinogens, bacteria, diabetes and fever as well as maintenance of proper cholesterol level of the body. Chili peppers are one of the richest sources of Vitamin C, Vitamin A and Vitamin B-6 or pyridoxine. Potassium, phosphorus, calcium and sulphur are the minerals present in it at higher amounts. With the presence of capsaicin, the fruit vegetable helps in opening up of sinuses, breaking up of mucus and dissolving of blood clots. It also helps in increasing the metabolic rate of the body. As a potential source, sometimes chilies also help in curing headaches and joint pains of the body.

Root vegetables

Among the root vegetables, radish, turnip, carrots and beets are used as medicinal vegetables preventing the body from various disorders. Radish helps in curing whooping cough, rheumatism, tuberculosis and asthma. Sometimes, radish also acts as an anti-viral agent. The leaves are very rich source of Vitamin C and A as well as minerals such as calcium, phosphorus, sodium and potassium.

Turnips on the other hand are a rich source of Vitamin C, pyridoxine and folic acid and some of the minerals like calcium, magnesium, and potassium. The major role played by turnip in human body is to help in blood purification and production of blood cells. Turnip leaves are high in iodine and the root helps in lowering the lipid level of the body and fight against infectious diseases. Other medicinal benefits of turnip also include growth and strengthening of bones and prevention of diabetes and as a memory booster.

The presence of beta-carotene in carrots helps in the maintenance of good vision, curing rheumatism, diseases of lungs, stomach, kidney and intestines and coughs. Consumption of carrots also helps in leveling cholesterol in the blood as well as fight against lung cancer.

Beet is generally a perfect cure for the people suffering from liver dys-functioning. Having very rich amount of iron, the green leaves of beet are helpful against anemia and also improves the flow of bile in the stomach. Beets also have anti-parasitic properties.

Bulb vegetables

Among bulb vegetables, onion and garlic are considered as medicines to cure various types of diseases ranging from less harmful to highly dangerous. Both of bulb crops add to vegetables in order to add flavor to the dish. In addition to be used as a flavoring agent, onion has anti-cardiac properties, helps in reducing the growth of fungus on the external body. In addition to Vitamin C, onion also contains minerals such as sulfur and chromium in appreciable quantities. Both of these crops have anti-cancerous properties and also help in strengthening the immune system of the body. The presence of sulfur provides many health benefits such as maintenance the sugar, cholesterol and blood pressure level in the blood. On the other hand garlic helps in recovering from throat and kidney problems, heart diseases as well as rheumatism. Garlic is, sometimes also consumed as an appetizer.

Green leafy and salad vegetables

It is well said the consumption of green vegetables is similar to consuming blood directly owing to their importance in human body and their requirements as well. Green vegetables are rich sources of Vitamin A, Vitamin B1, B2 and B6, Folic acid, Vitamin E, and Vitamin K. Minerals such as iron, calcium, magnesium and potassium are also present in these leaves. Green leafy vegetables are required for proper functioning of the nervous system of the body while these also contribute to reducing the stress as well as cancer causing agents. Dark green leaves also act as an antioxidant to reduce allergies and other inflammations. Leaves of some of the root vegetables such as beet and radish are also consumed that provides ample nutrition to carry on the various processes of the body. Beet, spinach and lettuce are very rich sources of Vitamin A and help in strengthening the vision. Leaves of lettuce, parsley and celery are consumed raw as salad and are very rich sources of Vitamin C and Vitamin A. Celery has medicinal properties to level blood pressure, protection from cancer causing agents, especially cigarette smoke, arthritis and anxiety. Parsley, on the other hand has medicinal benefits against bladder stones, flatulence, rheumatism, some microbes, high blood pressure and urinary tract infections.

Legumes

Legumes are one of the best sources of Proteins for vegetarians Beans help in reducing cholesterol level of the body, manage stress and fight with cancer causing agents. Other medicinal benefits of adding beans in the daily diet are regulation of blood sugar level and insulin level of the body. In addition to proteins, legumes are good sources of fiber, folic acid and Vitamins helping in prevention of stomach related problems such as constipation and gall stone. The ample amount of minerals is also present in legumes help in protecting the body from osteoporosis and other bone related problems.

Cucurbitaceous vegetables and fruits

The main vegetables under cucurbits include cucumber, pumpkin, watermelon, muskmelon, gourds, and squashes. All these vegetables are full of nutrients and medicinal values. Water is also one of the major components present in cucurbits in large quantity. Medicinal values of all these cucurbits are detailed in the next section.

Pumpkin and squashes

Pumpkin helps in curbing appetites, preventing strokes and also reduction in absorption of fats and calories. The seeds of this fruit are also used to control intestinal worms. Both pumpkin and squashes are a rich source of Vitamin A and minerals such as potassium, calcium and phosphorus as well.

Water melon and musk melon

Watermelon contains appreciable quantities of lycopene that helps in reducing the clotting of blood, colon cancer and prostate infection and asthma. With the presence of more than 95% of water, it is a very good source of lowering thirst during scorch summers. The medicinal properties of this fruit include anti-cancerous, anti-oxidant, and anti-bacterial that helps in blocking attacks of various microbes. Muskmelon also has varied medicinal properties that range of protection against skin problems to cancer. Other benefits of consuming muskmelon also include protection against diabetes, heart diseases, ulcers, urinary tract infections and formation of stones in the kidney.

Cucumber

Like watermelons, cucumbers also contain high amount of water hence best for people living in sandy regions. It cools of the body and help reduce body heat during summers. Cucumbers also contain fibers that help in easy digestion, and regulation of blood pressure. The fruit also helps in protecting skin and hair, overcoming bad breaths, reducing weight and reducing cholesterol.

Gourds

Bottle gourd, bitter gourd, snake gourd, round gourd, ivy gourd and wax gourd are some of the main vegetables that come under this category. One benefit of consuming gourds is that almost all the parts of these can be used for the treatment of varied ranges of diseases. Similar to their names, these gourds protect the body from the attack of various diseases and disorders. Consuming bottle gourd in cooked form helps in controlling diarrhea, diabetes, urinary disorders, ulcers and indigestion. While the decoction of leaves also helps in curing flatulence, the seeds of the vegetable are used to treat painful gums and toothache. The syrup of the fruit is used to treat colon related problems and fever.

All parts of bitter gourd can be used as medicines. The decoction of bitter gourd is used to control dysentery, fever, and treatments for arthritis, diabetes, constipation, hypertension, asthma, rheumatism and kidney stones. Sometime this vegetable also helps in curing skin related diseases. This bitter vegetable is the cure of diseases that range from normal to harmful such as cancer as the decoction of bitter gourd also helps in the treatment of cancer and inflammation of the colon.

Wax gourd is used against fever, inflammations, pains, respiratory disorders, and nervous disorders of the body. It also helps in preventing diabetes, diseases related to the kidneys and urinary problems. The roots of this vine are used to treat gonorrhea.

Sponge gourds are consumed to treat dysentery, asthma, gonorrhea, uterus disorders, jaundice, and smallpox and even in cancer too. The leaves of the plant are used against dysentery, headaches, swelling and rashes due to heat at the same helps in cooling the body.

Cole crops
Cole crops that include cabbage, cauliflower, broccoli, Brussels sprouts and knoll khol also have medicinal properties that protect the body from various diseases the major being cancers, high cholesterol and pregnancy and digestion related problems. Cabbage is an anti-oxidant that helps in neutralizing the effect of free radicals in the body. Cabbage is also considered as a good source of Vitamin A and Vitamin C along with minerals like calcium, phosphorous and potassium. Calcium in the vegetables helps in reducing inflammation of the joints however it is advised to patients suffering from goiter, to consult a physician before consuming these vegetables. Cabbage also prevents colon, stomach and breast cancers and the juice also helps in curing ulcers. Cauliflowers on the other hand help in protecting the body from uncontrolled growth of cells causing cancer especially breast and colon cancer. Like cabbage, broccoli also has high nutritive

24

value that works as an anti-oxidant, prevention against lung cancer, breast cancer, and colon cancer. Other medicinal benefits of consumption of broccoli in daily routine are that it helps in healing ulcers and sometimes also shows anti-viral activities. Another important vegetable among Cole crops is Brussels sprouts that are one of the excellent sources of Vitamin C and Vitamin A. It helps in detoxification of the body by facilitating activation of detoxification enzymes and also strengthens the immune system. The high content of Vitamin C present in Brussels sprouts also helps in the manufacturing of collagen[5] proteins

Conclusion

It is very important to have regular intake of vegetable in our daily diet to remain always protected from the attack of various diseases and disorders. A proper diet contains a good amount of vegetables and of various types as excess of one vegetables and lack of another may also cause deleterious effects. All nutrients are essential for the body to carry out our normal metabolic processes and almost all the nutrients are combined with each other either directly or indirectly to produce synergistic effect hence absence or deficiency of any of the nutrients effect the functioning of other related nutrients too. Vegetables are the only sources where more than one nutrients are present in appreciable amount thus, accepted and balanced intake of vegetables is utmost requirement of the body in order to lead a disease free healthy life.

---

[5] In animals, it is the main structural and abundant protein in the body

Annexure

Table 8: Vegetables as medicines to cure diseases

S.N	Diseases	Vegetables to be consumed
1	Acne	Vegetables rich in Vitamin A and Vitamin B-complex
2	Alzheimer's disease	Vegetables rich in Vitamin E, Vitamin B-complex and Zinc,
3	Anemia	Green leafy vegetables, beams and legumes
4	Anxiety	Green leafy vegetables, Vegetables rich in Vitamin B-complex and Calcium
5	Arthritis	Vegetables rich in Sulphur such as garlic, onion, asparagus and cabbage, Vitamin B complex and minerals such as Copper, Zinc and Selenium
6	Asthma	Yellow and green vegetables, garlic, onion, Vegetables rich in Vitamin C, and magnesium
7	Bad breathe	Salad vegetables, vegetables rich in Vitamin C such as peppers, spinach, cabbage and broccoli
8	Brain attack or stroke	Vegetables rich in dietary fibers, antioxidants and Vitamin B-complex
9	Bronchitis	Vegetables rich in Vitamin C and Vitamin E, garlic, ginger, and onions
10	Burns	Vegetables rich in Vitamin C, Vitamin A, Vitamin E, antioxidants and water
11	Cancer	Vegetables rich in dietary fibers, legumes, cole crops, fruit vegetables such as tomatoes and peppers, bulb crops and carrots
12	Cataract	Vegetables rich in anti-oxidants, carotenoids, Vitamin C and Vitamin E and Vitamin B-complex
13	Cholesterol	Vegetables rich in fibers, and Vitamin B3. Other vegetables to be consumed also include garlic and legumes
14	Constipation	Vegetables rich in dietary fibers, and magnesium
15	Common cold	Vegetables rich in Vitamin C, Zinc.
16	Dehydration	Vegetables rich in water especially cucurbits
17	Depression	Vegetables rich in Vitamin B-complex
18	Diabetes	Vitamin rich in Vitamin B complex, Vitamin E and Magnesium
19	Diarrhea	Vegetables rich in vitamins and water
20	Dysplasia	Vegetables rich in Vitamin B-complex, Vitamin C, Carotene and Calcium
21	Ear infections	Vegetables rich in Vitamin C
22	Eczema	Vegetables rich in anti-oxidants, fibers and Zinc
23	Flu	Vegetables rich in Vitamin C, legumes, garlic
24	Gall stones	Vegetables rich in fibers and Vitamin C and beets
25	Glaucoma	Vegetables rich in Vitamin C and magnesium
26	Goiter	Vegetables rich in Iodine

27	Gout	Vegetables rich in Vitamin C,
28	Gum diseases	Vegetables rich in Vitamin C, Vitamin E, Vitamin B-complex and Calcium
29	Heart failure	Vegetables rich in Vitamin B1, Calcium and Magnesium
30	Hyperactivity disorders	Vegetables such as amaranth and legumes, vegetables rich in Vitamin B-complex, Vitamin C, Magnesium, Iron, and Zinc
31	Hypertension	Vegetables such as garlic and legumes, vegetables rich in Potassium, Magnesium, Calcium and Vitamin C
32	Hypoglycemia	Vegetables rich in Vitamin B-complex, Vitamin C, dietary fibers and magnesium
33	Kidney stones	All green leafy vegetables, legumes, vegetables rich in Vitamin B6, Potassium, Calcium and Magnesium
34	Memory loss	Vegetables rich in Vitamin E and Vitamin B-complex
35	Osteoporosis	Vegetables rich in Calcium, Magnesium, Vitamin D and Vitamin K
36	Stress	Vegetables rich in Vitamin B-complex, Vitamin C, Calcium and Magnesium,
37	Ulcers	Vegetables rich in Vitamin K and Zinc

Source: Encyclopedia of Natural Cures

Table 9: Recommended amounts of daily vegetables intake

S.N	Amount of vegetables to be consumed on daily basis
Man (19-50 years)	3 cups
Woman (19-50 years)	2.5 cups
Boy (9-18 years)	2.5 to 3 cups
Girl (9-18 years)	2 to 2.5 cups
Child (2-8 years)	1 to 1.5 cups
Man (>51 years)	2.5 cups
Woman (>51 years)	2 cups

Source: http://www.choosemyplate.gov/food-groups/vegetables-amount.html

Table 10: Percentage of water, carbohydrate and proteins present in vegetables

S.N	Vegetable	Water (%)	Proteins (gm)	Calories	Dietary fiber (gm)
1	Amaranth	86	2.79	28	-
2	Artichoke	77	3.47	64	10.3
3	Asparagus	93	2.16	20	1.8
4	Beetroot	88	1.43	37	1.7

5	Brinjal	92	0.82	35	2.5
6	Broccoli	91	1.86	27	2.6
7	Brussels sprouts	86	3.98	56	4.1
8	Butternut squash	86	1.84	82	-
9	Cabbage	93	0.95	17	1.4
10	Capsicum	92	0.64	15	1.3
11	Carrot	87	0.59	27	2.3
12	Cauliflower	92	1.14	14	1.4
13	Celery	95	1.25	27	2.4
14	Chinese Broccoli	92	1	19	2.2
15	Chinese cabbage	95	1.78	17	2
16	Cucumber	96	0.34	8	0.3
17	French bean	92	12.48	228	16.6
18	Kale	91	2.47	36	2.6
19	Leek	79	1	38	1.2
20	Lima beans	67	14.66	216	13.2
21	Muskmelon	93	0.58	23	0.6
22	Okra	90	3	35	4
23	Onion	87	0.82	26	0.8
24	Peas	79	8.58	134	8.8
25	Potatoes	79	4.33	161	3.8
26	Pumpkin	92	1.76	49	2.7
27	Dakin Radish	94	0.98	25	2.4
28	Radish	95	0.39	9	0.9
29	Spinach	92	0.86	7	0.7
30	Summer squash	94	1.87	41	2
31	Sweet potatoes	68	2.29	103	3.8
32	Tomato	94	1.08	22	1.5
33	Turnip	92	1.11	34	3.1
34	Watermelon	92	1.74	86	1.1
35	Winter squash	88	1.82	76	5.7

Source: http://ndb.nal.usda.gov/ndb/search/list

Notes to study the table
- *Quantity of vitamins in 1/2 cup of vegetables- Asparagus, beet, broccoli, cabbage, carrots, cauliflower, cucumber, radish*
- *Quantity of vitamin present in medium size of Artichoke, potato, sweet potato, musk melon, tomato and small size of capsicum and onion*
- *Rest of the figures- Quantity of vitamins in 1 cup of vegetables*

Table 11: Common vegetables and percentage of vitamin present-1

S. N	Vegetables	Vitamin A (IU)	Vitamin C (mg)	Vitamin E (mg)	Vitamin K (mcg)
1	Alfalfa	51	2.7	0.01	10.1
2	Amaranth	3656	54.3	-	-
3	Artichoke	16	8.9	0.23	17.8
4	Asparagus	905	6.9	1.35	45.5
5	Beetroot	30	3.1	0.03	0.2
6	Brinjal	37	1.3	0.41	2.9
7	Broccoli	1207	50.6	1.13	110
8	Brussels sprouts	1209	96.7	0.67	218.9
9	Butternut squash	22868	31	2.64	2
10	Cabbage	60	28.1	0.11	81.5
11	Capsicum	274	59.5	0.27	5.5
12	Carrot	13286	2.8	0.8	10.7
13	Cauliflower	7	27.5	0.04	8.6
14	Celery	782	9.2	0.53 IU	56.7
15	Chinese Broccoli	1441	24.8	0.42	74.6
16	Chinese cabbage	1151	18.8	-	-
17	Cucumber	55	1.5	0.02	8.5
18	French bean	5	2.1	-	-
19	Kale	17,707	53.3	1.1	1062
20	Leek	1007	5.2	0.62	31.5
21	Lima beans	-	-	0.34	3.8
22	Muskmelon	2334	25.3	0.03	1.7
23	Okra	453	26.1	0.43	64
24	Onion	1	3.1	0.01	0.3
25	Peas	1282	22.7	0.22	41.4
26	Potatoes	17	16.6	0.07	3.5
27	Pumpkin	12230	11.5	1.96	2
28	Dakin Radish	-	22.2	-	0.4
29	Radish	4	8.6	-	0.8
30	Spinach	2813 mg	8.4	0.61	144.9
31	Summer squash	2011 mg	20.9	0.22	7.9
32	Sweet potatoes	21,909mg	22.3	0.81	2.6
33	Tomato	1025	15.6	0.66	9.7
34	Turnip	-	18.1	0.03	0.2
35	Watermelon	1627	23.2	0.14	0.3
36	Winter squash	10707 mg	19.7	0.25	9

Source: http://ndb.nal.usda.gov/ndb/search/list

Notes to study the table
- *Quantity of vitamins in 1/2 cup of vegetables- Asparagus, beet, broccoli, cabbage, carrots, cauliflower, cucumber, radish*
- *Quantity of vitamin present in medium size of Artichoke, potato, sweet potato, musk melon, tomato and small size of capsicum and onion*
- *Rest of the figures- Quantity of vitamins in 1 cup of vegetables*

Table 12: Common vegetables and percentage of vitamin present-2

S.N	Vegetables	VitB1 (mg)	VitB2 (mg)	VitB3 (mg)	VitB5 (mg)	VitB6 (mg)	Folate (mcg)
1	Alfalfa	0.03	0.04	0.159	0.186	0.011	12
2	Amaranth	0.03	0.18	0.738	0.082	0.234	75
3	Artichoke	0.06	0.11	1.332	0.288	0.097	107
4	Asparagus	0.15	0.13	0.976	0.203	0.071	134
5	Beetroot	0.02	0.03	0.281	0.123	0.057	68
6	Brinjal	0.08	0.02	0.594	0.074	0.085	14
7	Broccoli	0.05	0.10	0	0.48	0.156	84
8	Brussels sprouts	0.17	0.13	0.947	0.393	0.278	94
9	Butternut squash	0.15	0.04	1.986	0.736	0.254	39
10	Cabbage	0.05	0.03	0.186	0.13	0.084	22
11	Capsicum	0.04	0.02	0.355	0.073	0.166	7
12	Carrot	0.05	0.03	0.503	0.181	0.119	11
13	Cauliflower	0.03	0.03	0.254	0.315	0.107	27
14	Celery	0.06	0.07	0.479	0.292	0.129	33
15	Chinese Broccoli	0.08	0.13	0.385	0.14	0.062	87
16	Chinese cabbage	0.05	0.05	0.595	0.095	0.0211	63
17	Cucumber	0.01	0.02	0.051	0.135	0.021	4
18	French bean	0.23	0.11	0.966	0.393	0.186	133
19	Kale	0.07	0.09	0.65	0.064	0.179	17
20	Leek	0.03	0.03	0.248	0.089	0.14	30
21	Lima beans	0.30	0.10	0.791	0.793	0.303	156
22	Musk melon	0.028	0.013	0.506	0.072	0.05	14
23	Okra	0.21	0.09	1.394	0.341	0.299	74
24	Onion	0.03	0.01	0.099	0.068	0.077	9
25	Peas	0.41	0.24	3.234	0.245	0.346	101
26	Potatoes	0.11	0.08	2.439	0.65	0.538	48
27	Pumpkin	0.08	0.19	1.012	0.492	0.108	22
28	Dakin Radish	-	0.034	0.221	0.168	0.056	25
29	Radish	0.007	0.023	0.147	0.096	0.041	14
30	Spinach	0.023	0.057	0.217	0.02	0.059	58
31	Summer squash	0.077	0.045	.913	0.581	0.14	41
32	Sweet potatoes	0.122	0.121	1.695	1.008	0.326	7
33	Tomato	0.046	0.023	0.731	0.109	0.098	18
34	Turnip	0.042	0.036	0.466	0.222	0.105	14

35	Water melon	0.094	0.06	0.509	0.632	0.129	9
36	Winter squash	0.033	0.137	1.015	0.48	0.33	41

Source: http://ndb.nal.usda.gov/ndb/search/list

Notes to study the table

- *Quantity of vitamins in 1/2 cup of vegetables- Asparagus, beet, broccoli, cabbage, carrots, cauliflower, cucumber, radish*
- *Quantity of vitamin present in medium size of Artichoke, potato, sweet potato, musk melon, tomato and small size of capsicum and onion*
- *Rest of the figures- Quantity of vitamins in 1 cup of vegetables*

Table 13 Percentage of minerals present in vegetables

Vegetables	Ca (mg)	Cu (mg)	Iron (mg)	Mg (mg)	Mn (mg)	P (mg)	K (mg)	Se (mcg)	Na (mg)	Zn (mg)
Alfalfa	11	0.052	0.32	9	0.062	23	26	0.2	2	0.3
Amaranth	276	0.209	2.98	73	1.137	95	846	1.2	28	1.16
Artichoke	25	0.152	0.73	50	0.27	88	343	0.2	72	0.48
Asparagus	21	0.149	0.82	13	0.139	49	202	5.5	13	0.54
Beetroot	14	0.063	0.67	20	0.277	32	259	0.6	65	0.3
Brinjal	6	0.058	0.25	11	0.112	15	122	0.1	1	0.12
Broccoli	31	0.048	0.52	16	0.151	52	229	1.2	32	0.35
Chinese broccoli	88	0.054	0.49	16	0.232	36	230	1.1	6	0.34
Brussels sprouts	56	0.129	1.87	31	0.354	87	495	2.3	33	0.51
Butternut squash	84	0.133	1.23	59	0.353	55	582	1	8	0.27
Cabbage	36	0.013	0.13	11	0.154	25	147	0.5	6	0.15
Capsicum	7	0.049	0.25	7	0.09	15	130	-	2	0.1
Carrot	23	0.052	0.27	8	0.062	23	183	0.2	5	0.3
Cauliflower	10	0.011	0.2	6	0.082	20	88	0.4	9	0.11
Celery	63	0.054	0.63	18	0.159	38	426	1.5	136	0.21
Chinese cabbage	38	0.035	0.36	12	0.182	46	268	0.5	11	0.21
Cucumber	8	0.021	0.15	7	0.041	12	76	0.2	1	0.1
French bean	112	0.204	1.91	99	0.676	181	655	2.1	11	1.13
Kale	94	0.203	1.17	23	0.541	36	296	1.2	30	0.31
Leek	37	0.077	1.36	17	0.306	21	108	0.6	12	0.07
Lima beans	32	0.442	4.49	81	0.97	209	955	-	4	1.79
Muskmelon	6	0.028	0.14	8	0.028	10	184	0.3	11	0.12
Okra	123	0.136	0.45	58	0.47	51	216	0.6	10	0.69
Onion	13	0.0	0.1	7	0.092	21	100	0.4	2	0.13

		4	4							
Peas	43	0.277	2.46	62	0.84	187	434	-	5	1.9
Potatoes	26	0.204	1.87	48	0.379	121	926	0.7	17	0.62
Pumpkin	37	0.223	1.4	22	0.218	74	564	0.5	2	0.56
Dakin Radish	25	0.148	0.22	13	0.049	35	419	1	19	0.19
Radish	14	0.029	0.2	6	0.04	12	135	0.3	23	0.16
Spinach	30	0.039	0.81	24	0.269	15	167	0.3	24	0.16
Summer squash	40	0.117	0.67	29	0.283	52	319	-	2	0.4
Sweet potatoes	43	0.184	0.79	31	0.567	62	542	-	41	0.36
Tomato	12	0.073	0.33	14	0.14	30	292	-	6	0.21
Turnip	51	0.003	0.28	14	0.111	41	276	0.3	25	0.19
Watermelon	20	0.12	0.69	29	0.109	31	320	1.1	3	0.29
Winter squash	45	0.168	0.9	27	0.383	39	494	0.8	2	0.45

Source: http://ndb.nal.usda.gov/ndb/search/list

Ca- Calcium, Cu- Copper, Mg- Magnesium, Mn- Manganese, P- Phosphorous, K- Potassium, Se- Selenium, Na- Sodium, Zn- Zinc

Notes to study the table
- *Quantity of vitamins in 1/2 cup of vegetables- Asparagus, beet, broccoli, cabbage, carrots, cauliflower, cucumber, radish*
- *Quantity of vitamin present in medium size of Artichoke, potato, sweet potato, musk melon, tomato and small size of capsicum and onion*
- *Rest of the figures- Quantity of vitamins in 1 cup of vegetables*

Bibliography

Choudhary, B. (1992). *Vegetables* . New Delhi : National Book Trust of India

Sherry Torkos, B.Sc. (2008). The Canadian Encyclopedia of Natural Medicine. Canada: Tri-Graphic Printing, Ltd.

United States Department of Agriculture